The Ultimate Bread Machine Cooking Guide For Beginners

Simple And Delicious Bread Maker Recipes

Jude Lamb

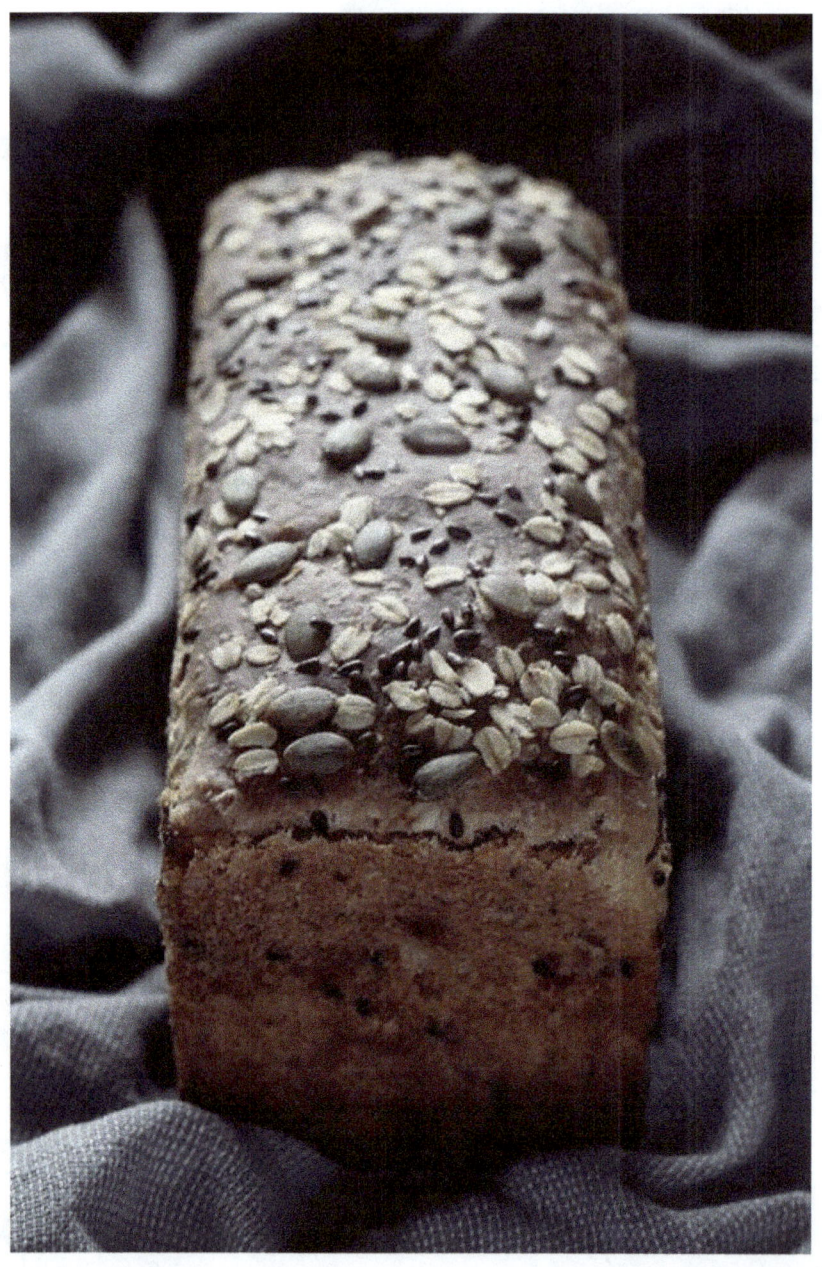

© Copyright 2020 - All rights reserved.

The content contained within this book may not be reproduced, duplicated or transmitted without direct written permission from the author or the publisher.

Under no circumstances will any blame or legal responsibility be held against the publisher, or author, for any damages, reparation, or monetary loss due to the information contained within this book. Either directly or indirectly.

Legal Notice:

This book is copyright protected. This book is only for personal use. You cannot amend, distribute, sell, use, quote or paraphrase any part, or the content within this book, without the consent of the author or publisher.

Disclaimer Notice:

Please note the information contained within this document is for educational and entertainment purposes only. All effort has been executed to present accurate, up to date, and reliable, complete information. No warranties of any kind are declared or implied. Readers acknowledge that the author is not engaging in the rendering of legal, financial, medical or professional advice. The content within this book has been derived from various sources. Please consult a licensed professional before attempting any techniques outlined in this book.

By reading this document, the reader agrees that under no circumstances is the author responsible for any losses, direct or indirect, which are incurred as a result of the use of information contained within this document, including, but not limited to, — errors, omissions, or inaccuracies.

Table of contents

Making Bread 7

French Cheese Bread 9

Beer Cheese Bread 11

Jalapeno Cheese Bread 13

Cheddar Cheese Bread 15

Cottage Cheese and Chive Bread 18

Ricotta Bread 20

Oregano Cheese Bread 22

Spinach and Feta Bread 24

Italian Cheese Bread 27

Onion, Garlic, Cheese Bread 29

Cream Cheese Bread 31

Mozzarella Cheese and Salami Loaf 33

Olive and Cheddar Loaf 36

Cottage Cheese Bread 39

Green Cheese Bread 41

Cheesy Chipotle Bread 44

Cheddar Cheese Basil Bread 46

Olive Cheese Bread 48

Double Cheese Bread 50

Chile Cheese Bacon Bread	53
Italian Parmesan Bread	56
Feta Oregano Bread	58
Awesome Rosemary Bread	60
Original Italian Herb Bread	62
Lovely Aromatic Lavender Bread	65
Cinnamon & Dried Fruits Bread	67
Herbal Garlic Cream Cheese Delight	70
Oregano Mozza-Cheese Bread	72
Cumin Tossed Fancy Bread	75
Potato Rosemary Loaf	77
Delicious Honey Lavender Bread	80
Inspiring Cinnamon Bread	82
Lavender Buttermilk Bread	84
Cajun Bread	86
Turmeric Bread	88
Rosemary Cranberry Pecan Bread	90
Sesame French Bread	93
Garlic, Herb, and Cheese Bread	95
Savoury Herb Blend Bread	97
Semolina Bread	100
Seeded Bread	103

Macadamia Bread 105

Orangey Almond Bacon Bread 107

Making Bread

There is nothing like the scent of freshly baked bread to greet you when you wake up. Bakers traditionally produced their products during the early hours meaning their loaves were fresh, hot, and mouth-watering tasty for hungry customers wanting a slice of bread to go with a slap-up breakfast.

Bread historically dates back to Neolithic or even prehistoric times in its earliest incarnation.

Prime ingredients include flour and water used to make the dough. The dough can have numerous additives to offer assorted consistency, flavors, and healthy preferences. Additives may include yeast, fat, salt, baking soda, fruits, spices, eggs, milk, sugar, or vegetables. You can even add seeds to the bread, oils, and nuts. Bread is quite a versatile product and can be devoured on its own or as an accompaniment to the main dish. The dough is traditionally baked, but modern alternatives could include steaming.

The outer part of the bread, commonly known as the crust, can be baked into a hard or soft version. The inner part of the bread is classed as the "crumb," strangely not the small bits that cover your lap.

The prime time to eat a loaf of bread is soon after it has been removed from the oven. At this delicious time, the bread is warm, aromatic, and fresh. Leaving the bread for any length of time will cause the bread to become stale.

A quirk dating back to the 13th century was the Baker's Dozen.

A Baker's Dozen, ironic as it was from the 13th century, relates to 13 items making a dozen instead of the usual 1 1/2. As history would have us believe, a Baker's dozen suggested that punishment was administered to bakers who short-changed their customers. One way to ensure that a customer always received a full quota was to give more bread than paid for. Furthermore, if one loaf was damaged, burnt or was of unacceptable quality, there were still 1 1/2 loaves available for the customer.

Another explanation of the Baker's Dozen, and slightly more believable, is that when round loaves were placed on a standard baking tray, the configuration was 3+2+3+2+3 which gave a greater density to the tray and allowed easier stacking.

Over the decades, the baking of bread has followed the path of many traditions updated to reflect the changing needs of society. Whereas bread was always the preserve of the local baker, modern supermarkets now have their own "in-house" ovens, and bread is baked to suit customer demand.

French Cheese Bread

Preparation Time: 5 minutes

1½-Pound Loaf

Ingredients:

- 1 teaspoon sugar
- 2¼ teaspoons yeast
- 1¼ cups water
- 3 cups bread flour
- 2 tablespoons parmesan cheese
- 1 teaspoon garlic powder
- 1½ teaspoons salt

Directions:

1. Add each ingredient to the bread machine in the order and at the temperature recommended by your bread machine manufacturer.
2. Close the lid, select the basic bread, medium crust setting on your bread machine, and press start.

3. When the bread machine has finished baking, remove the bread and put it on a cooling rack.

Nutrition:

- Carbohydrates: 21 g
- Fat: 6 g
- Protein: 1½ g
- Calories: 170
- Sodium: 240 mg

Beer Cheese Bread

Preparation Time: 5 minutes

1½-Pound Loaf

Ingredients:

- 1 package active dry yeast
- 3 cups bread flour
- 1 tablespoon sugar
- 1½ teaspoons salt
- 1 tablespoon room temperature butter
- 1¼ cup room temperature beer
- ½ cup shredded or diced American cheese
- ½ cup shredded or diced Monterey jack cheese

Directions:

1. Heat the beer and American cheese in the microwave together until just warm.
2. Add each ingredient to the bread machine in the order and at the temperature recommended by your bread machine manufacturer.

3. Close the lid, select the basic bread, medium crust setting on your bread machine and press start.

4. When the bread machine has finished baking, remove the bread and put it on a cooling rack.

Nutrition:

- Calories: 180
- Carbohydrates: 21 g
- Fat: 5 g
- Protein: 5 g
- Sodium: 360 mg

Jalapeno Cheese Bread

Preparation Time: 5 minutes

1-Pound Loaf

Ingredients:

- 3 cups bread flour
- 1½ teaspoons active dry yeast
- 1 cup water
- 2 tablespoons sugar
- 1 teaspoon salt
- ½ cup shredded cheddar cheese
- ¼ cup diced jalapeno peppers

Directions:

1. Add each ingredient to the bread machine in the order and at the temperature recommended by your bread machine manufacturer.
2. Close the lid, select the basic bread, medium crust setting on your bread machine, and press start.

3. When the bread machine has finished baking, remove the bread and put it on a cooling rack.

Nutrition:

- Calories: 185
- Carbohydrates: 22 g
- Fat: 4 g
- Protein: 7 g
- Calories: 150
- Sodium: 290 mg

Cheddar Cheese Bread

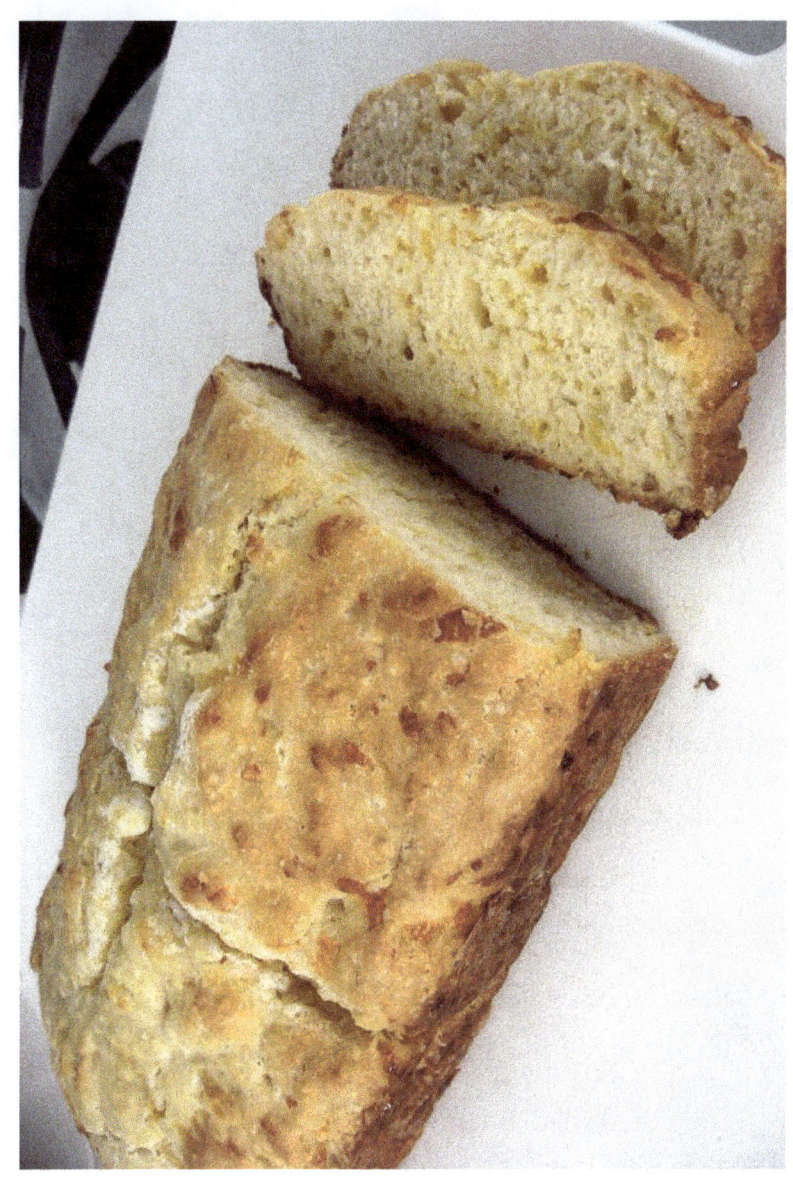

Preparation Time: 5 minutes

1-Pound Loaf

Ingredients:

- 1 cup lukewarm milk
- 3 cups all-purpose flour
- 1¼ teaspoons salt
- 1 teaspoon tabasco sauce, optional
- ¼ cup Vermont cheese powder
- 1 tablespoon sugar
- 1 cup grated cheddar cheese, firmly packed
- 1½ teaspoons instant yeast

Directions:

1. Add each ingredient to the bread machine in the order and at the temperature recommended by your bread machine manufacturer.
2. Close the lid, select the basic bread, medium crust setting on your bread machine, and press start.
3. When the bread machine has finished baking, remove the bread and put it on a cooling rack.

Nutrition:

- Calories: 182
- Carbohydrates: 25 g
- Fat: 4 g Protein: 7 g
- Sodium: 300mg

Cottage Cheese and Chive Bread

Preparation Time: 5 minutes

3-Pound Loaf

Ingredients:

- 3½ cups water
- 1 cup cottage cheese
- 1 large egg
- 2 tablespoons butter
- 1½ teaspoons salt
- 3¾ cups white bread flour
- 3 tablespoons dried chives
- 2½ tablespoons granulated sugar
- 2¼ teaspoons active dry yeast

Directions:

1. Add each ingredient to the bread machine in the order and at the temperature recommended by your bread machine manufacturer.
2. Close the lid, select the basic bread, medium crust setting on your bread machine, and press start.

3. When the bread machine has finished baking, remove the bread and put it on a cooling rack.

Nutrition:

- Calories: 196
- Carbohydrates: 33 g
- Fat: 4 g Protein: 7 g
- Sodium 320 mg

Ricotta Bread

Preparation Time: 5 minutes

1-Pound Loaf

Ingredients:

- 3 tablespoons skim milk
- ¼ cup water
- 2/3 cups ricotta cheese
- 4 teaspoons unsalted butter, softened to room temperature
- 1 large egg
- 2 tablespoons granulated sugar
- ½ teaspoon salt
- 1½ cups bread flour, + more flour, as needed
- 1 teaspoon active dry yeast

Directions:

1. Add each ingredient to the bread machine in the order and at the temperature recommended by your bread machine manufacturer.

2. Close the lid, select the basic bread, medium crust setting on your bread machine, and press start.

3. When the bread machine has finished baking, remove the bread and put it on a cooling rack.

Nutrition:

- Calories: 174
- Carbohydrates: 3 g
- Fat: 1½ g
- Protein: 11 g
- Sodium: 120 mg

Oregano Cheese Bread

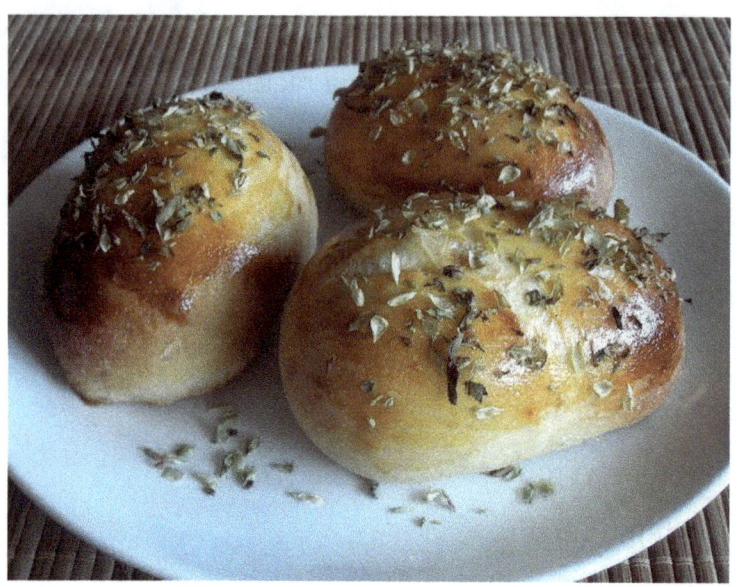

Preparation Time: 5 minutes

1-Pound Loaf

- **Ingredients:**
- 3 cups bread flour
- 1 cup water
- ½ cup freshly grated parmesan cheese
- 3 tablespoons sugar
- 1 tablespoon dried leaf oregano

- 1½ tablespoons olive oil
- 1 teaspoon salt
- 2 teaspoons active dry yeast

Directions:

1. Add each ingredient to the bread machine in the order and at the temperature recommended by your bread machine manufacturer.
2. Close the lid, select the basic bread, medium crust setting on your bread machine, and press start.
3. When the bread machine has finished baking, remove the bread and put it on a cooling rack.

Nutrition:

- Calories: 184
- Carbohydrates: 22 g
- Fat: 5 g
- Protein: 3 g
- Sodium: 240 mg

Spinach and Feta Bread

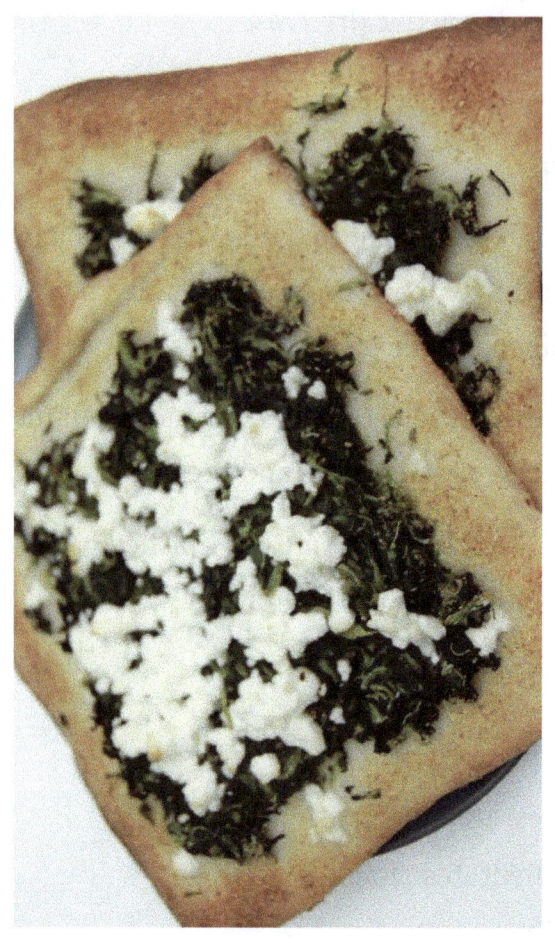

Preparation Time: 5 minutes

1-Pound Loaf

Ingredients:

- 1 cup water
- 2 teaspoons butter
- 3 cups flour
- 1 teaspoon sugar
- 2 teaspoons instant minced onion
- 1 teaspoon salt
- 1¼ teaspoons instant yeast
- 1 cup crumbled feta
- 1 cup chopped fresh spinach leaves

Directions:

1. Add each ingredient except the cheese and spinach to the bread machine in the order and at the temperature recommended by your bread machine manufacturer.
2. Close the lid, select the basic bread, medium crust setting on your bread machine, and press start.
3. When only 5 minutes are left in the last kneading cycle add the spinach and cheese.
4. When the bread machine has finished baking, remove the bread and put it on a cooling rack.

Nutrition:

- Calories: 184
- Carbohydrates: 5g
- Fat: 6 g
- Protein: 6 g
- Sodium: 240 mg

Italian Cheese Bread

Preparation Time: 5 minutes

1½-Pound Loaf

Ingredients:

- 1¼ cup water
- 3 cups bread flour
- ½ shredded pepper jack cheese
- 2 teaspoons Italian seasoning
- 2 tablespoons brown sugar
- 1½ teaspoons salt
- 2 teaspoons active dry yeast

Directions:

1. Add each ingredient to the bread machine in the order and at the temperature recommended by your bread machine manufacturer.
2. Close the lid, select the basic bread, medium crust setting on your bread machine, and press start.

3. When the bread machine has finished baking, remove the bread and put it on a cooling rack.

Nutrition:

- Calories: 180
- Carbohydrates: 1g
- Fat: 6 g
- Protein: 7 g
- Sodium: 350 mg

Onion, Garlic, Cheese Bread

Preparation Time: 10 minutes

1½-Pound Loaf

Ingredients:

- 3 tablespoons dried minced onion
- 3 cups bread flour
- 2 teaspoons garlic powder
- 2 teaspoons Active dry yeast
- 2 tablespoons white sugar
- 2 tablespoons margarine
- 2 tablespoons dry milk powder
- 1 cup shredded sharp cheddar cheese
- 1½ cups warm water
- 1½ teaspoons salt

Directions:

1. In the order suggested by the manufacturer, put the flour, water, powdered milk, margarine or butter, salt, and yeast in the bread pan.

2. Press the basic cycle with a light crust. When the manufacturer directs the sound alerts, add two teaspoons of the onion flakes, the garlic powder, and shredded cheese.

3. After the last kneed, sprinkle the remaining onion flakes over the dough.

Nutrition:

- Total Fat: 6 g
- Carbohydrates: 29
- Protein: 12 g
- Sodium: 380 mg

Cream Cheese Bread

Preparation Time: 10 minutes

1 Pound- Loaf

Ingredients:

- ½ cup water
- ½ cup cream cheese, softened
- 2 tablespoons melted butter
- 1 beaten egg
- 4 tablespoons sugar
- 1 teaspoon salt
- 3 cups bread flour
- 1½ teaspoons active dry yeast

Directions:

1. Place the ingredients in the pan in order, as suggested by your bread machine.
2. After removing it from a machine, place it in a greased 9x5 pound pan after the cycle.
3. Cover and let rise until doubled.

4. Bake in a 350° F oven for approximately 35 minutes.

Nutrition:

- Carbohydrates: 24 g
- Total Fat: 5 g
- Protein: 3 g
- Sodium: 240 mg

Mozzarella Cheese and Salami Loaf

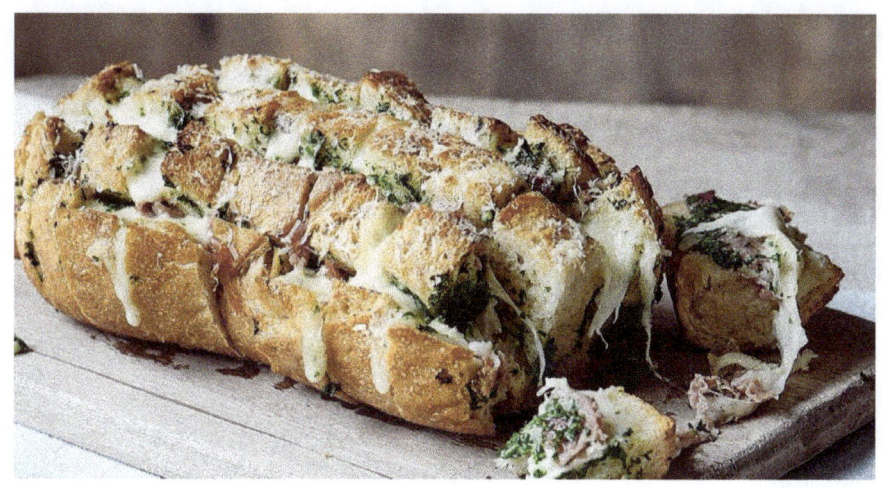

Preparation Time: 20 minutes

1-Pound Loaf

Ingredients:

- ¾ cup water
- 1/3 cup mozzarella cheese, shredded
- 4 teaspoons sugar
- 2/3 teaspoon salt
- 2/3 teaspoon dried basil

- Pinch of garlic powder
- 2 cups + 2 tablespoons white bread flour
- 1 teaspoon instant yeast
- ½ cup hot salami, finely diced

Directions:

1. Add the listed ingredients to your bread machine (except salami), following the manufactures instructions.
2. Set the bread machine's program to Basic/White Bread and the crust type to light. Press Start.
3. Let the bread machine work and wait until it beeps. This is your indication to add the remaining ingredients at this point, add the salami.
4. Wait until the remaining bake cycle completes.
5. Once the pound is done, take the bucket out from the bread machine and let it rest for 5 minutes.
6. Gently shake the bucket and remove the pound, transfer the pound to a cooling rack, and slice.
7. Serve and enjoy!

Nutrition:

- Calories: 214
- Carbohydrates: 22 g
- Total Fat: 3 g
- Protein: 6 g
- Sugar: 2 g
- Sodium: 350 mg

Olive and Cheddar Loaf

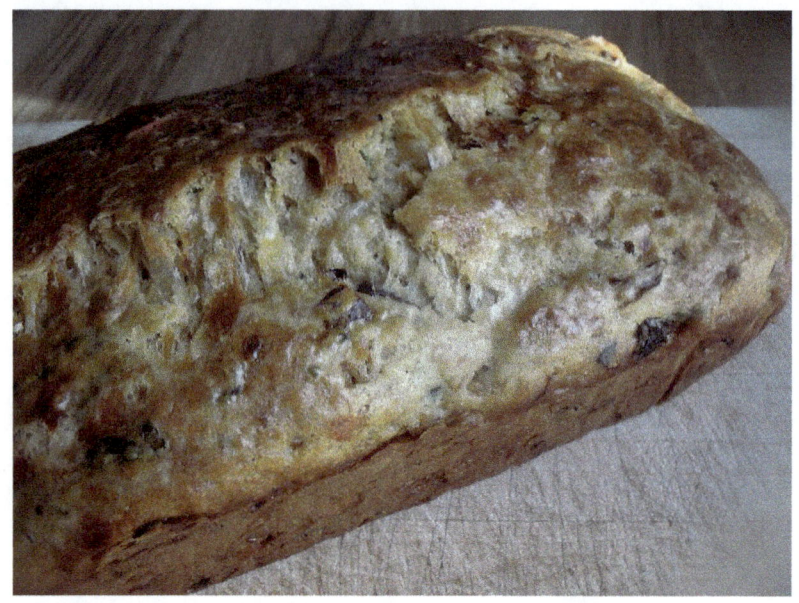

Preparation Time: 20 minutes

1-Pound Loaf

Ingredients:

- 1 cup water, room temperature
- 4 teaspoons sugar
- ¾ teaspoon salt
- 1 cup sharp cheddar cheese, shredded

- 3 cups bread flour
- 2 teaspoons active dry yeast
- ¾ cup pimiento olives, drained and sliced

Directions:

1. Add the listed ingredients to your bread machine (except salami), following the manufactures instructions.
2. Set the bread machine's program to Basic/White Bread and the crust type to light. Press Start.
3. Let the bread machine work and wait until it beeps. This is your indication to add the remaining ingredients. At this point, add the salami.
4. Wait until the remaining bake cycle completes.
5. Once the pound is done, take the bucket out from the bread machine and let it rest for 5 minutes.
6. Gently shake the bucket and remove the pound, transfer the pound to a cooling rack, and slice.
7. Serve and enjoy!

Nutrition:

- Calories: 190 Carbohydrates: 19 g
- Total Fat: 4 g Protein: 5 g
- Sugar: 5 g Sodium: 300 mg

Cottage Cheese Bread

Preparation Time: 2 hours 50 minutes

Cooking Time: 15 minutes

1-Pound loaf

Ingredients:

- ½ cup water
- 1 cup cottage cheese
- 2 tablespoons margarine
- 1 egg
- 1 tablespoon white sugar
- ¼ teaspoon baking soda
- 1 teaspoon salt
- 3 cups bread flour
- 2 ½ teaspoons active dry yeast

Directions:

1. Into the bread machine, place the ingredients according to the manufacturer's order, then push the start button. In case the dough looks too sticky, feel free to use up to half a cup more bread flour.

2. Gently shake the bucket and remove the pound, transfer the pound to a cooling rack, and slice.

3. Serve and enjoy

Nutrition:

- Calories: 191
- Carbohydrates: 26 g
- Cholesterol: 11mg
- Total Fat: 3.6 g
- Protein: 7.3 g
- Sodium: 384 mg

Green Cheese Bread

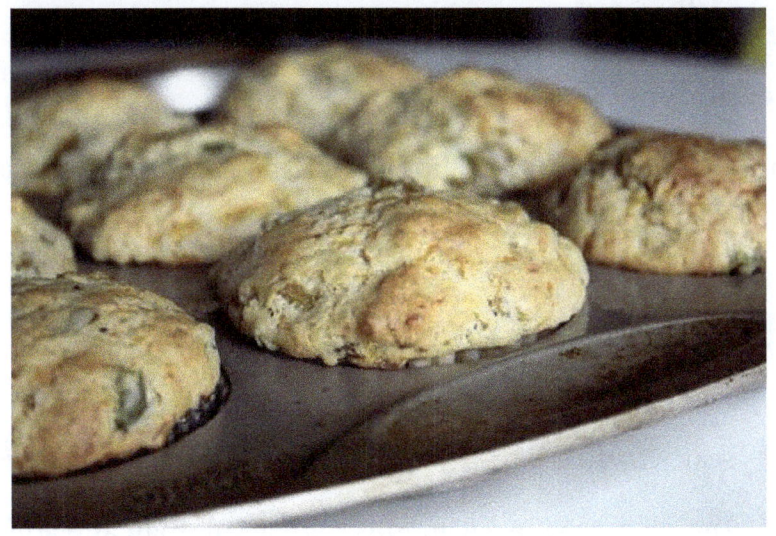

Preparation Time: 1 hour

1-Pound Loaf

Ingredients:

- ¾ cup lukewarm water
- 1 tablespoon sugar
- 1 teaspoon kosher salt
- 2 tablespoons green cheese
- 1 cup of wheat bread machine flour
- 5 cups whole-grain flour, finely ground

- 1 teaspoon bread machine yeast
- 1 teaspoon ground paprika

Directions:

1. Place all the dry and liquid ingredients, except paprika, in the pan and follow the instructions for your bread machine.
2. Pay particular attention to measuring the ingredients. Use a measuring cup, measuring spoon, and kitchen scales to do so.
3. Dissolve yeast in warm milk with a saucepan and add in the last turn.
4. Add paprika after the beep or place it in the dispenser of the bread machine.
5. Set the baking program to BASIC and the crust type to DARK.
6. If the dough is too wet, adjust the recipe's amount of flour and liquid.
7. When the program has ended, take the pan out of the bread machine and cool for 5 minutes.
8. Shake the pound out of the pan. If necessary, use a spatula.

9. Wrap the bread with a kitchen towel and set it aside for an hour. Otherwise, you can cool it on a wire rack.

Nutrition:

- Calories: 181
- Carbohydrates: 23.6 g
- Cholesterol: 2 g
- Total Fat: 1 g
- Protein: 4.1 g
- Sodium: 304 mg
- Sugar: 1.6 g

Cheesy Chipotle Bread

Preparation Time: 20 minutes

1-Pound Loaf

Ingredients:

- 2/3 cup water, 80°F
- 1½ tablespoons sugar
- 1½ tablespoons powdered skim milk
- ¾ teaspoon salt
- ½ teaspoon chipotle chili powder
- 2 cups white bread flour
- ½ cup (2 ounces) shredded sharp Cheddar cheese
- ¾ teaspoon instant yeast

Directions:

1. Place the ingredients in your machine as recommended on it.
2. Make a program on the machine for basic white Bread, select Light or medium crust, and press Start.

3. When the pound is finished, remove the bucket from the machine.

4. Let the pound cool for 5 minutes.

5. Gently shake the bucket and remove the pound and turn it out onto a rack to cool.

Nutrition:

- Calories: 189
- Carbohydrates: 27 g
- Total Fat: 1 g
- Protein: 6 g
- Sodium: 245 m

Cheddar Cheese Basil Bread

Preparation Time: 2 hours

1-Pound Loaf

Ingredients:

- 2/3 cup milk, set at 80°F
- 2 teaspoons melted butter, cooled
- 2 teaspoons sugar
- 2/3 teaspoon dried basil
- ½ cup (2 ounces) shredded sharp Cheddar cheese
- ½ teaspoon salt
- 2 cups white bread flour
- 1 teaspoon active dry yeast.

Directions:

1. Place the ingredients in your machine as recommended on it.
2. Make a Program on the machine for basic white Bread, select Light or medium crust, and press Start.

3. When the pound is finished, remove the bucket from the machine.

4. Let the pound cool for 5 minutes.

5. Gently shake the bucket and remove the pound and turn it out onto a rack to cool.

Nutrition:

- Calories: 170
- Carbohydrates: 26 g
- Total Fat: 4 g
- Protein: 6 g
- Sodium: 130 mg

Olive Cheese Bread

Preparation Time: 15 minutes

Ingredients:

- 2/3 cup milk, set at 80°F
- 1 tablespoon melted butter cooled
- 2/3 teaspoon minced garlic
- 1 tablespoon sugar
- 2/3 teaspoon salt
- 2 cups white bread flour
- ½ cup (2 ounces) shredded Swiss cheese
- ¾ teaspoon bread machine or instant yeast
- ¼ cup chopped black olives

Directions:

1. Place the ingredients in your device as recommended on it.
2. Make a program on the machine for basic white Bread, select Light or medium crust, and press Start.
3. When the pound is finished, remove the bucket from the machine.

4. Let the pound cool for 5 minutes.

5. Gently shake the bucket and remove the pound and turn it out onto a rack to cool.

Nutrition:

- Calories: 175
- Carbohydrates: 27 g
- Total Fat: 5 g
- Protein: 6 g
- Sodium: 260 mg

Double Cheese Bread

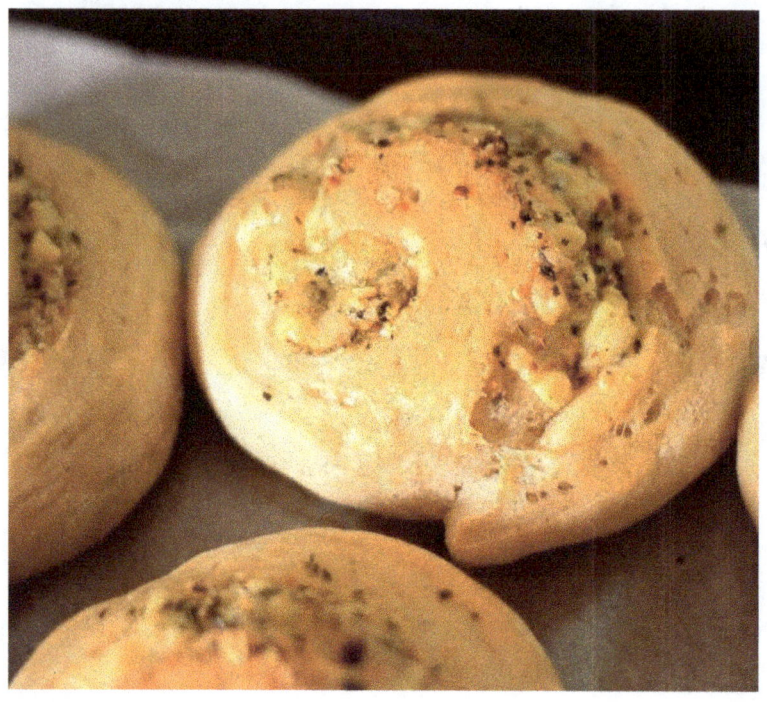

Preparation Time: 2 hours

1-Pound Loaf

Ingredients:

- ¾ cup plus 1 tablespoon milk
- 2 teaspoons butter, melted and cooled
- 4 teaspoons sugar

- 2/3 teaspoon salt
- 1/3 teaspoon freshly ground black pepper
- Pinch cayenne pepper
- 1 cup (4 ounces) shredded aged sharp Cheddar cheese
- 1/3 cup shredded or grated Parmesan cheese
- 2 cups white bread flour
- ¾ teaspoon instant yeast

Directions:

1. Place the ingredients in your machine as recommended on it.
2. Make a program on the machine for Basic White bread, select light or medium crust, and press Start.
3. When the pound is finished, remove the bucket from the machine.
4. Let the pound cool for 5 minutes.
5. Gently shake the bucket and remove the pound and turn it out onto a rack to cool.

Nutrition:

- Calories: 183
- Carbohydrate: 21 g
- Total Fat: 4g
- Protein: 6 g
- Sodium: 244 mg

Chile Cheese Bacon Bread

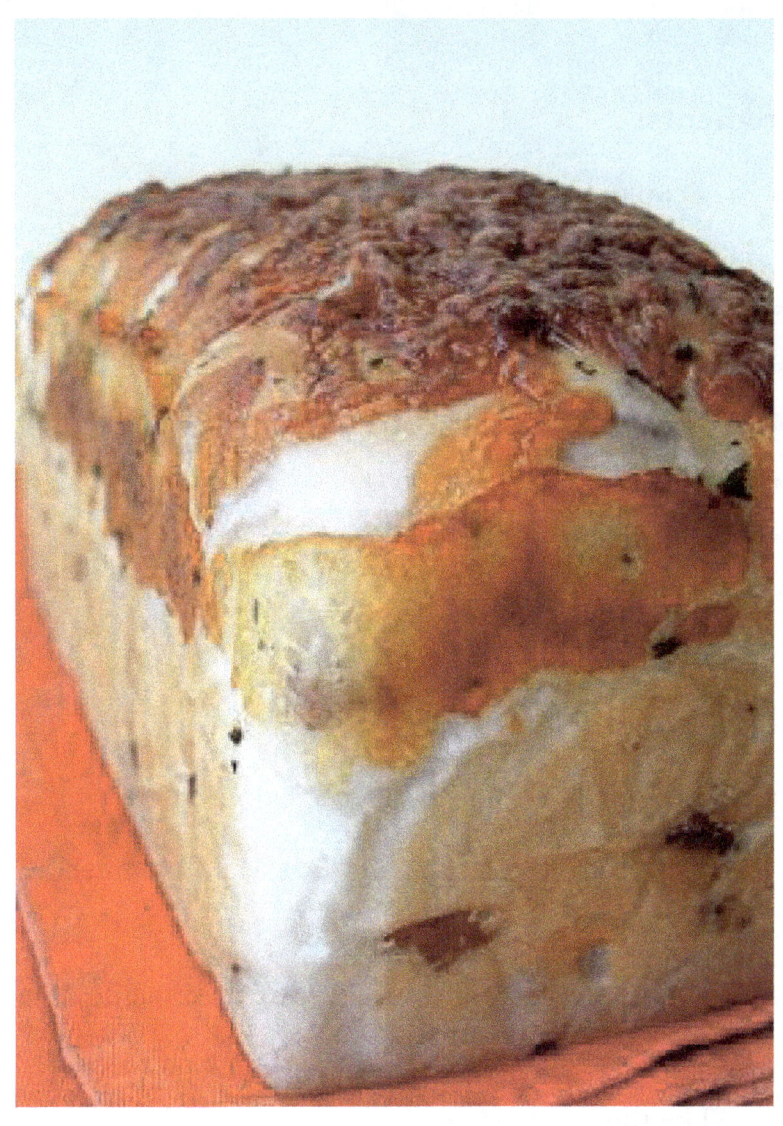

Preparation Time: 15 minutes

1-Pound Loaf

Ingredients:

- 1/3 cup milk
- 1 teaspoon melted butter cooled
- 1 tablespoon honey
- 1 teaspoon salt
- 1/3 cup chopped and drained green Chile
- 1/3 cup grated Cheddar cheese
- 1/3 cup chopped cooked bacon
- 2 cups white bread flour
- 11/3 teaspoons bread machine or instant yeast

Directions:

1. Place the ingredients in your device as recommended on it.
2. Make a program on the machine for basic white Bread, select Light or medium crust, and press Start.
3. When the pound is finished, remove the bucket from the machine.
4. Let the pound cool for 5 minutes.

5. Gently shake the bucket and remove the pound and turn it out onto a rack to cool.

Nutrition

- Calories: 174
- Carbohydrates: 40 g
- Total Fat: 4 g
- Protein: 6 g
- Sodium: 240 mg

Italian Parmesan Bread

Preparation Time: 5 minutes

1-Pound Loaf

Ingredients:

- ¾ cup water
- 2 tablespoons melted butter
- 2 teaspoons sugar
- 2/3 teaspoon salt
- 11/3 teaspoons chopped fresh basil
- 2 2/3 tablespoons grated Parmesan cheese
- 2 1/3 cups white bread flour
- 1 teaspoon bread machine or instant yeast

Directions:

1. Place the ingredients in your device as recommended on it.
2. Make a program on the machine for Basic White bread, select light or medium crust, and press Start.
3. When it's finished, remove the bucket from the machine.

4. Let the pound cool for 5 minutes.

5. Gently shake the bucket and remove the pound and turn it out onto a rack to cool.

Nutrition:

- Calories: 171
- Carbohydrates: 29 g
- Total Fat: 4 g
- Protein: 5 g
- Sodium: 237 mg

Feta Oregano Bread

Preparation Time: 15 minutes

1-Pound Loaf

Ingredients:

- 2/3 cup of milk, at 80°F
- 2 teaspoons melted butter, cooled
- 2 teaspoons sugar
- 2/3 teaspoon salt
- 2 teaspoons dried oregano
- 2 cups white bread flour
- 1½ teaspoons bread machine or instant yeast
- 2/3 cup (2½ ounces) crumbled feta cheese

Directions:

1. Place the ingredients in your device as recommended on it.
2. Make a program on the machine for Basic White bread, select light or medium crust, and press Start.
3. When it's finished, remove the bucket from the machine.

4. Let the pound cool for 5 minutes.
5. Gently shake the bucket and remove the pound and turn it out onto a rack to cool.

Nutrition:

- Calories: 170
- Carbohydrates: 27 g
- Fat: 4g
- Protein: 5
- Sodium: 180 mg

Awesome Rosemary Bread

Preparation Time: 15 minutes

1 ½-Pound Loaf

Ingredients:

- ¾ cup + 1 tablespoon water
- 12/3 tablespoons melted butter, cooled
- 2 teaspoons sugar
- 1 teaspoon salt
- 1 tablespoon fresh rosemary, chopped
- 2 cups white bread flour
- 11/3 teaspoons instant yeast

Directions:

1. Combine all of the ingredients to your bread machine, carefully following the instructions of the manufacturer.
2. Set the program of your bread machine to Basic/White Bread and set crust type to Medium.
3. Press START.
4. Wait until the cycle completes.

5. Once the pound is ready, take the bucket out and allow the pound to chill for 5 minutes.

6. Gently jiggle the bucket to take out the pound.

Nutrition:
- Carbohydrates: 25g
- Fiber: 1g
- Protein: 4g
- Fat: 3g
- Calories: 1270
- Sodium: 240 mg

Original Italian Herb Bread

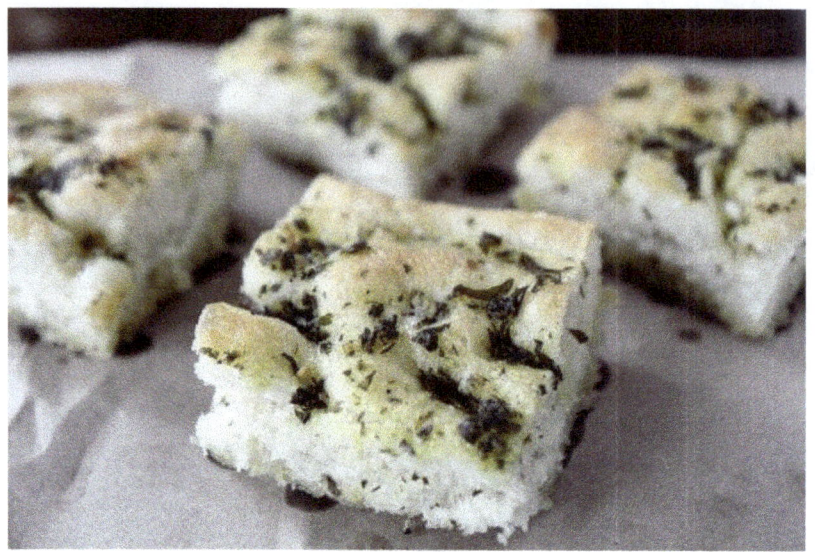

Preparation Time: 15 minutes

1½-Pound Loaf

Ingredients:

- 1 cup water
- ½ cup olive brine
- 1½ tablespoons butter
- 3 tablespoons sugar

- 2 teaspoons salt
- 51/3 cups flour
- 2 teaspoons bread machine yeast
- 1 olive, black/green
- 1½ teaspoons Italian herbs

Directions:

1. Cut olives into pounds.
2. Put all ingredients into your bread machine (except olives), carefully following the instructions of the manufacturer.
3. Set the program of your bread machine to French bread and set crust type to Medium.
4. Once the maker beeps, add olives.
5. Wait until the cycle completes.
6. Once the pound is ready, take the bucket out and cool the pound for 5 minutes.
7. Wobble the bucket to take off the pound.

Nutrition:

- Calories. 180 Carbohydrates: 21 g
- Fiber: 1g Fat: 7g
- Protein: 1g Sodium: 320 mg

Lovely Aromatic Lavender Bread

Preparation Time: 15 minutes

1-Pound Loaf

Ingredients:

- ¾ cup milk
- 1 tablespoon melted butter, cooled
- 1 tablespoon sugar
- ¾ teaspoon salt
- 1 teaspoon fresh lavender flower, chopped
- ¼ teaspoon lemon zest
- ¼ teaspoon fresh thyme, chopped
- 2 cups white bread flour
- ¾ teaspoon instant yeast

Directions:

1. Add all of the ingredients to your bread machine, carefully following the instructions of the manufacturer.

2. Set the program of your bread machine to Basic/White Bread and set crust type to Medium.

3. Wait until the cycle completes.

4. Once the pound is ready, take the bucket out and let the pound cool for 5 minutes.

5. Gently shake the bucket to remove the pound.

Nutrition:

- Calories: 160
- Carbohydrates: 27 g
- Fiber: 1 g
- Protein: 4 g
- Fat: 2 g
- Sodium: 180 mg

Cinnamon & Dried Fruits Bread

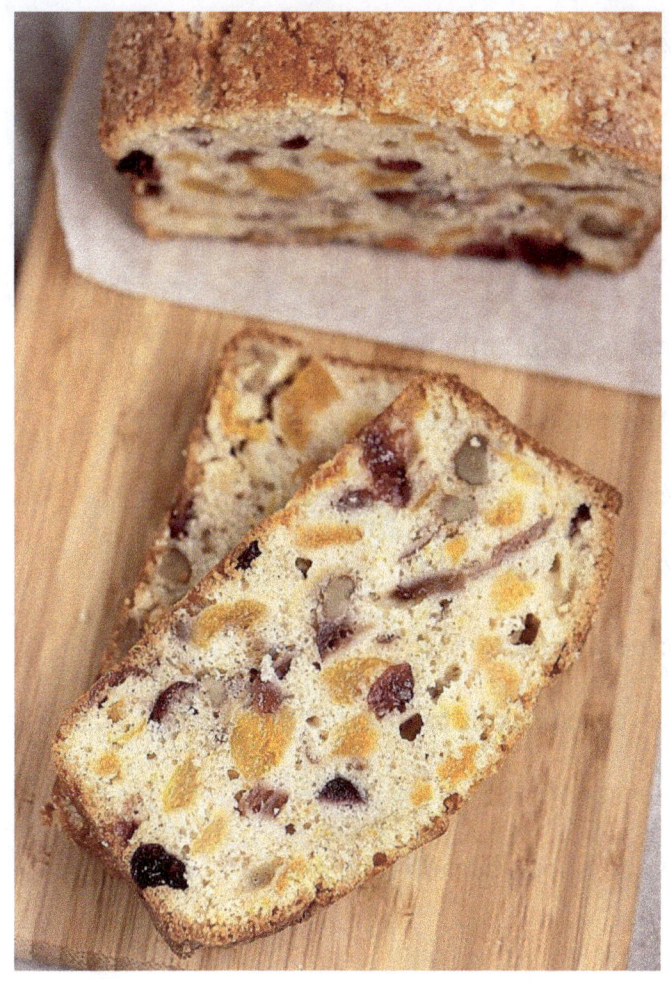

Preparation Time: 20 minutes

1-Pound Loaf

Ingredients:

- 2¾ cups flour
- ¾ cup water
- 1½ cups dried fruits
- 4 tablespoons sugar
- 2½ tablespoons butter
- 1 tablespoon milk powder
- 1 teaspoon cinnamon
- ½ teaspoon ground nutmeg
- ¼ teaspoon vanillin
- ½ cup peanuts
- powdered sugar, for sprinkling
- 1 teaspoon salt
- 1½ teaspoon bread machine yeast

Directions:

1. Add all of the ingredients to your bread machine (except peanuts and powdered sugar), carefully following the instructions of the manufacturer.

2. Set the program of your bread machine to Basic/White Bread and set crust type to Medium.
3. Once the bread maker beeps, moisten dough with a bit of water and add peanuts.
4. Wait until the cycle completes.
5. Once the pound is ready, take the bucket out and let the pound cool for 5 minutes.
6. Gently shake the bucket to remove the pound.
7. Sprinkle with powdered sugar.

Nutrition:

- Calories: 315
- Carbohydrates: 65 g
- Fiber: 1 g
- Protein: 5 g
- Fat: 4 g
- Sodium: 240 mg

Herbal Garlic Cream Cheese Delight

Preparation Time: 20 minutes

1-Pound Loaf

Ingredients:

- 1/3 cup water
- 1/3 cup herb and garlic cream cheese mix, at room temp
- 1 whole egg, beaten, at room temp
- 4 teaspoons melted butter, cooled
- 1 tablespoon sugar
- 2/3 teaspoon salt
- 2 cups white bread flour
- 1 teaspoon instant yeast

Directions:

1. Add all of the ingredients to your bread machine, carefully following the instructions of the manufacturer.
2. Set the program of your bread machine to Basic/White Bread and set crust type to Medium.

3. Wait until the cycle completes.
4. Once the pound is ready, take the bucket out and let the pound cool for 5 minutes.
5. Gently shake the bucket to remove the pound.

Nutrition:

- Calories:182
- Carbohydrates: 27 g
- Fiber: 2 g
- Protein: 5 g
- Fat: 6 g
- Sodium: 200 mg

Oregano Mozza-Cheese Bread

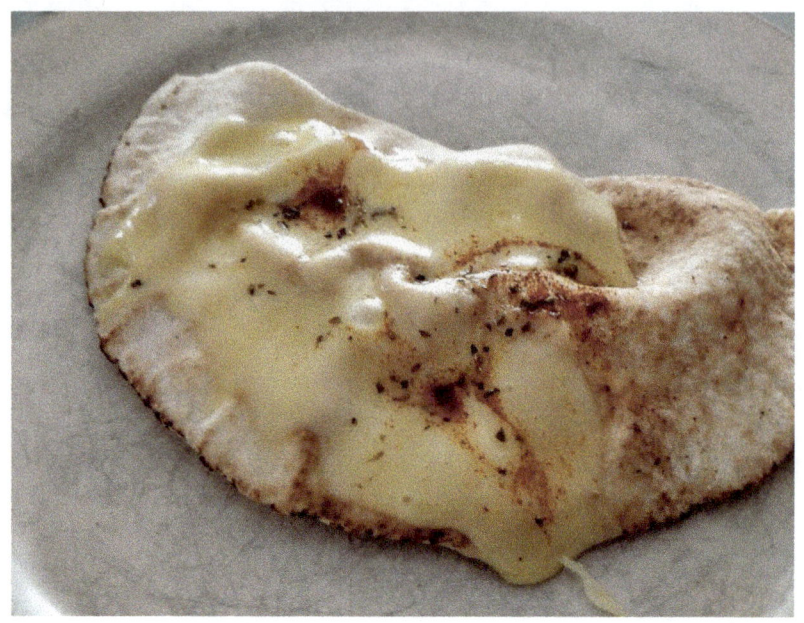

Preparation Time: 15 minutes

1 ½ -Pound loaf

Ingredients:

- 1 cup (milk + egg) mixture
- ½ cup mozzarella cheese
- 2¼ cups flour

- ¾ cup whole grain flour
- 2 tablespoons sugar
- 1 teaspoon salt
- 2 teaspoons oregano
- 1½ teaspoons dry yeast

Directions:

- Add all of the ingredients to your bread machine, carefully following the instructions of the manufacturer.
- Set the program of your bread machine to Basic/White Bread and set crust type to Dark.
- Wait until the cycle completes.
- Once the pound is ready, take the bucket out and let the pound cool for 5 minutes.
- Gently shake the bucket to remove the pound.

Nutrition:

- Calories: 190
- Carbohydrates: 40 g

- Fiber: 1g
- Protein: 7.7g
- Fat: 2.1g
- Sodium: 220 mg

Cumin Tossed Fancy Bread

Preparation Time: 10 minutes

2-Pound Loaf

Ingredients:

- 5 1/3 cups wheat flour
- 1½ teaspoons salt
- 1½ tablespoons sugar
- 1 tablespoon dry yeast
- 1¾ cups water
- 2 tablespoons cumin
- *3 tablespoons sunflower oil*

Directions:

1. Add warm water to the bread machine bucket.
2. Add salt, sugar, and sunflower oil.
3. Sift in wheat flour and add yeast.

4. Set the program of your bread machine to French bread and set crust type to Medium.

5. Once the maker beeps, add cumin.

6. Wait until the cycle completes.

7. Once the pound is ready, take the bucket out and let the pound cool for 5 minutes.

8. Gently shake the bucket to remove the pound.

Nutrition:

- Calories: 161
- Carbohydrates: 67 g
- Fiber: 2g
- Protein: 9.5g
- Fat: 7g
- Sodium: 220 mg

Potato Rosemary Loaf

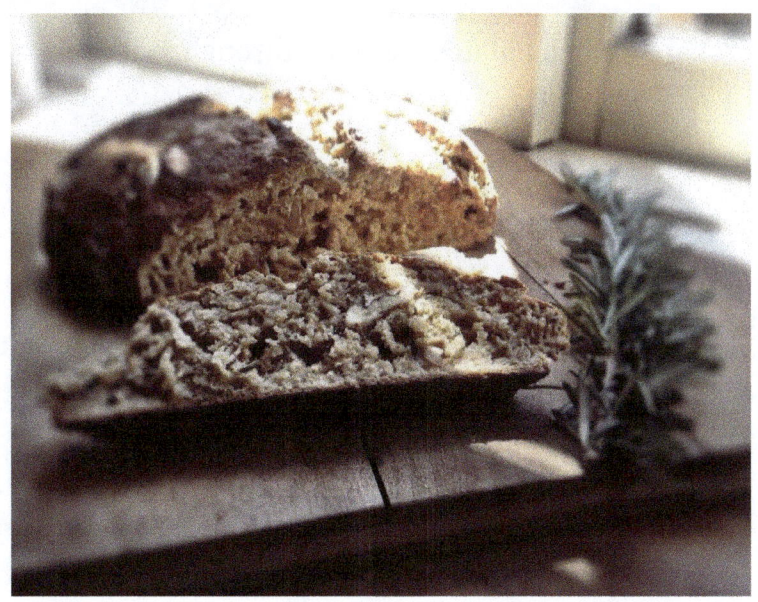

Preparation Time: 25 minutes

1½ Pound Loaf

Ingredients:

- 4 cups wheat flour
- 1 tablespoon sugar
- 1 tablespoon sunflower oil
- 1½ teaspoons salt

- 1½ cups water
- 1 teaspoon dry yeast
- 1 cup mashed potatoes, ground through a sieve
- crushed rosemary to taste

Directions:

- Add flour, salt, and sugar to the bread maker bucket and attach mixing paddle.
- Add sunflower oil and water.
- Put in yeast as directed.
- Set the program of your bread machine to Bread with Filling mode and set crust type to Medium.
- Once the bread maker beeps and signals to add more ingredients, open the lid, add mashed potatoes, and chopped rosemary.
- Wait until the cycle completes.
- Once the pound is ready, take the bucket out and let the pound cool for 5 minutes.
- Gently shake the bucket to remove the pound.

Nutrition:

- Calories: 276
- Carbohydrates: 54 g
- Fiber: 1 g
- Protein: 12 g
- Fat: 3g
- Sodium: 220 mg

Delicious Honey Lavender Bread

Preparation Time: 20 minutes
1½ Pound Loaf

Ingredients:

- 1½ cups wheat flour
- 21/3 cups whole meal flour
- 1 teaspoon fresh yeast
- 1½ cups water
- 1 teaspoon lavender
- 1½ tablespoons honey
- 1 teaspoon salt

Directions:

1. Sift both types of flour in a bowl and mix.
2. Add all of the ingredients to your bread machine, carefully following the instructions of the manufacturer.
3. Set the program of your bread machine to Basic/White Bread and set crust type to Medium.
4. Wait until the cycle completes.
5. Once the pound is ready, take the bucket out and let the pound cool for 5 minutes.
6. Gently shake the bucket to remove the pound.

Nutrition:

- Calories: 226
- Carbohydrates: 46 g
- Fiber: 1g
- Protein: 7.5g
- Fat: 1.5g
- Sodium: 240 mg

Inspiring Cinnamon Bread

Preparation Time: 15 minutes
1-Pound Loaf

Ingredients:

- 2/3 cup milk
- 1 whole egg, beaten
- 3 tablespoons melted butter, cooled
- 1/3 cup sugar
- 1/3 teaspoon salt
- 1 teaspoon ground cinnamon
- 2 cups white bread flour
- 1 1/3 teaspoons active dry yeast

Directions:

1. Add all of the ingredients to your bread machine, carefully following the instructions of the manufacturer.
2. Set the program of your bread machine to Basic/White Bread and set crust type to Medium.
3. Wait until the cycle completes.
4. Once the pound is ready, take the bucket out and let the pound cool for 5 minutes.
5. Remove the pound

Nutrition:

- Calories: 191
- Carbohydrates: 34 g
- Fiber: 1g
- Protein: 5g
- Fat: 5g
- Sodium: 60 mg

Lavender Buttermilk Bread

Preparation Time: 10 minutes

1½-Pound Loaf

Ingredients:

- ½ cup water
- ½ cup buttermilk
- ¼ cup olive oil
- 3 tablespoons finely chopped fresh lavender leaves
- 1 ¼ teaspoons finely chopped fresh lavender flowers
- grated zest of 1 lemon
- 4 cups bread flour
- 2 teaspoons salt
- 2 ¾ teaspoons bread machine yeast

Directions:

1. Add each ingredient to the bread machine in the order and at the temperature recommended by your bread machine manufacturer.
2. Close the lid, select the basic bread, medium crust setting on your bread machine, and press start.

3. When the bread machine has finished baking, remove the bread and put it on a cooling rack.

Nutrition:

- Calories: 175
- Carbohydrates: 27 g
- Fat: 5 g
- Protein: 2 g
- Calories: 170
- Sodium: 480 mg

Cajun Bread

Preparation Time: 10 minutes

1-Pound Loaf

Ingredients:

- ½ cup water
- ¼ cup chopped onion
- ¼ cup chopped green bell pepper
- 2 teaspoons finely chopped garlic
- 2 teaspoons soft butter
- 2 cups bread flour
- 1 tablespoon sugar
- 1 teaspoon Cajun
- ½ teaspoon salt
- 1 teaspoon active dry yeast

Directions:

1. Add each ingredient to the bread machine in the order and at the temperature recommended by your bread machine manufacturer.

2. Close the lid, select the basic bread, medium crust setting on your bread machine, and press start.

3. When the bread machine has finished baking, remove the bread and put it on a cooling rack.

Nutrition:

- Calories: 170
- Carbohydrates: 23 g
- Fat: 4 g
- Protein: 5 g
- Sodium: 120 mg

Turmeric Bread

Preparation Time: 10 minutes

1 ½-Pound Loaf

Ingredients:

- 1 teaspoon dried yeast
- 4 cups strong white flour
- 1 teaspoon turmeric powder
- 2 teaspoons beetroot powder
- 2 tablespoons olive oil
- 1½ teaspoons salt
- 1 teaspoon chili flakes
- 1½ cups water

Directions:

1. Add each ingredient to the bread machine in the order and at the temperature recommended by your bread machine manufacturer.
2. Close the lid, select the basic bread, medium crust setting on your bread machine, and press start.

3. When the bread machine has finished baking, remove the bread and put it on a cooling rack.

Nutrition:

- Calories: 172
- Carbohydrates: 24 g
- Fat: 3 g
- Protein: 2 g
- Sodium: 360 mg

Rosemary Cranberry Pecan Bread

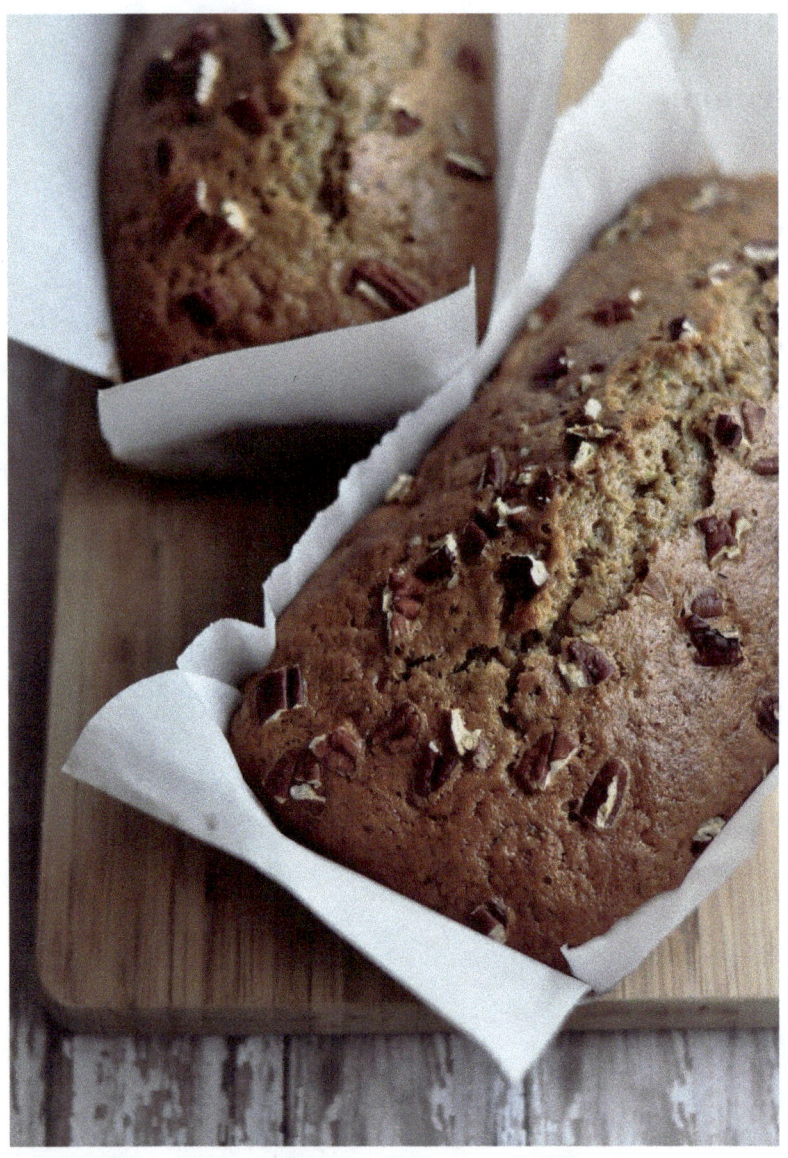

Preparation Time: 10 minutes

2-Pound Loaf

Ingredients:

- 1 1/3 cups water, plus
- 2 tablespoons water
- 2 tablespoons butter
- 2 teaspoons salt
- 4 cups bread flour
- ¾ cup dried sweetened cranberries
- ¾ cup toasted chopped pecans
- 2 tablespoons non-fat powdered milk
- ¼ cup sugar
- 2 teaspoons yeast

Directions:

1. Add each ingredient to the bread machine in the order and at the temperature recommended by your bread machine manufacturer.

2. Close the lid, select the basic bread, medium crust setting on your bread machine, and press start. When the bread machine has finished baking, remove the bread and put it on a cooling rack.

Nutrition:

- Calories: 171
- Carbohydrates: 12
- Fat: 5
- Protein: 9
- Sodium: 480 mg

Sesame French Bread

Preparation Time: 10 minutes

1½-Pound Loaf

Ingredients:

- 1½ cups water
- 1 tablespoon butter, softened
- 3 cups bread flour
- 2 teaspoons sugar
- 1 teaspoon salt
- 2 teaspoons yeast
- 2 tablespoons sesame seeds toasted

Directions:

1. Add each ingredient to the bread machine in the order and at the temperature recommended by your bread machine manufacturer.
2. Close the lid, select the French bread, medium crust setting on your bread machine, and press start.

3. When the bread machine has finished baking, remove the bread and put it on a cooling rack.

Nutrition:

- Calories: 165
- Carbohydrates: 21
- Fat: 3
- Protein: 6 g
- Sodium: 180 mg

Garlic, Herb, and Cheese Bread

Preparation Time: 20 minutes

1 ½-Pound Loaf

Ingredients:

- ½ cup ghee
- 6 eggs
- 2 cups almond flour
- 1 tablespoon baking powder
- ½ teaspoon Xanthan gum
- 1 cup cheddar cheese, shredded
- 1 tablespoon garlic powder
- 1 tablespoon parsley
- ½ tablespoon oregano
- ½ teaspoon salt

Directions:

1. Lightly beat eggs and ghee before pouring into the bread machine pan.
2. Add the remaining ingredients to the pan.

3. Set bread machine to gluten-free.

4. When the bread is finished, remove the bread pan from the bread machine.

5. Let it cool for a while before transferring it into a cooling rack.

6. You can store your bread for up to 5 days in the refrigerator.

Nutrition:
- Calories: 186
- Carbohydrates: 4 g
- Protein: 5 g
- Fat: 13 g
- Sodium: 120 mg

Savoury Herb Blend Bread

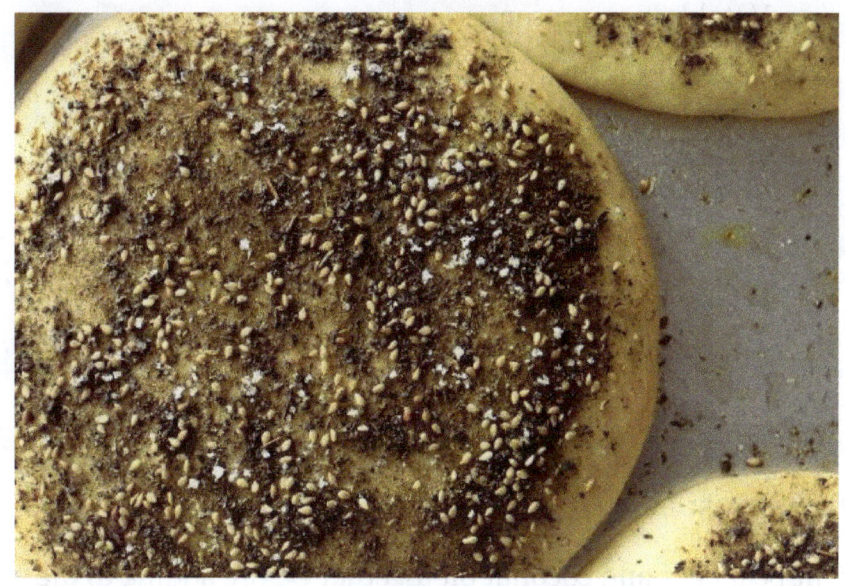

Preparation Time: 20 minutes

1½-Pound Loaf

Ingredients:

- 1 cup almond flour
- 1 cup water
- ½ cup coconut flour
- 1 cup parmesan cheese
- ¾ teaspoon baking powder

- 3 eggs
- 3 tablespoons coconut oil
- ½ tablespoon rosemary
- ½ teaspoon thyme, ground
- ½ teaspoon sage, ground
- ½ teaspoon oregano
- ½ teaspoon garlic powder
- ½ teaspoon onion powder
- ¼ teaspoon salt

Directions:

Light beat eggs and coconut oil together before adding to the bread machine pan.

Add all the remaining ingredients to the bread machine pan.

Set the bread machine to the gluten-free setting.

When the bread is finished, remove the bread machine pan from the bread machine.

Let cool slightly before transferring to a cooling rack.

You can store your bread for up to 7 days.

Nutrition:

- Calories: 180
- Carbohydrates: 6 g
- Protein: 9 g
- Fat: 15 g
- Sodium: 160 mg

Semolina Bread

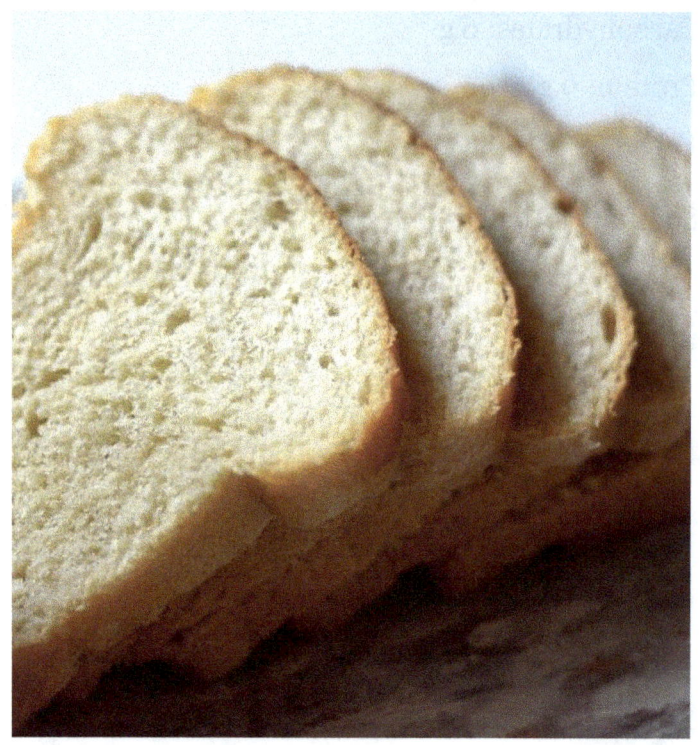

Preparation Time: 20 minutes

1-Pound Loaf

Ingredients:

- 1 cup almond fine flour
- 1 cup semolina flour

- 1 teaspoon yeast
- 1 egg
- 1 teaspoon salt
- 2 teaspoons Stevia powder
- 2 teaspoons Olive oil extra
- 1 cup warm water
- 2 teaspoons sesame seeds

Directions:

1. Get a mixing container and combine the almond flour, semolina flour, salt, and stevia powder.
2. In another mixing container, combine the egg, extra virgin olive oil, and warm water.
3. By instructions on your machine's manual, pour the ingredients in the bread pan, and follow how to mix in the yeast.
4. Put the bread pan in the machine, select the basic bread setting together with the bread size and crust type, if available, then press start once you have closed the machine's lid.
5. When the bread is ready, open the lid and spread the sesame seeds at the top, and close for a few minutes.

6. By using oven mitts, remove the pan from the machine. Use a stainless spatula to extract the pan's bread and turn the pan upside down on a metallic rack where the bread will cool off before slicing it.

Nutrition:

- Calories: 180
- Carbohydrates: 2.2 g
- Protein: 5g
- Fat: 1g
- Sodium: 200 mg

Seeded Bread

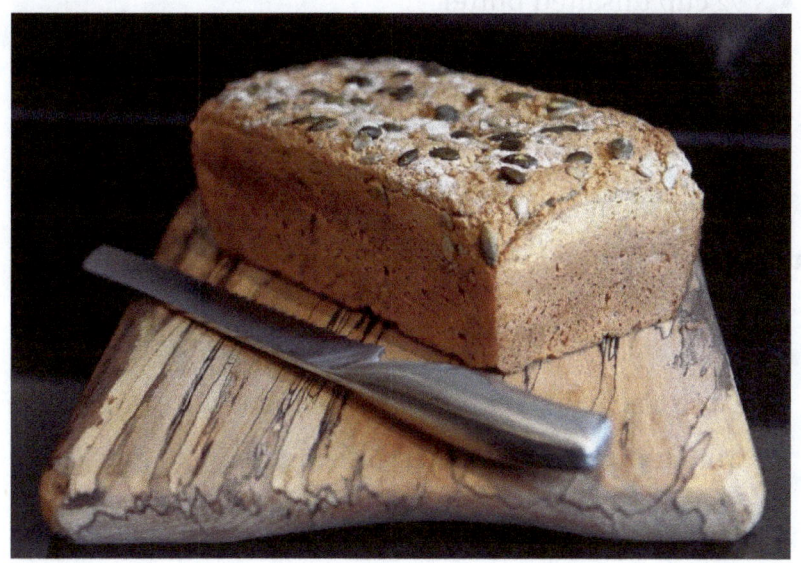

Preparation Time: 10 minutes

1-Pound Loaf

Ingredients:

- 2 tablespoons chia seeds
- ½ cup water
- ¼ teaspoon salt
- 7 large eggs

- ½ easpoon Xanthan gum
- 2 cups almond flour
- 1 teaspoon baking powder
- ½ cup unsalted butter
- 3 tablespoons sesame seeds
- 2 tablespoons olive oil

Directions:

1. Add all the ingredients to the Bread machine.
2. Close the lid and choose Bread mode. Once done, take out from the machine and cut into at least 5 pounds.
3. This seeded bread can be kept for up to 4-5 days in the fridge.

Nutrition:

- Calories: 190
- Fat: 4 g
- Carbohydrates: 4 g
- Protein: 6 g
- Sodium: 150 mg

Macadamia Bread

Preparation Time: 30 minutes

1-Pound Loaf

Ingredients:

- ¼ cup almond flour
- ½ cup water
- 1 cup macadamia nuts
- 2 tablespoons flax meal
- 1 teaspoon baking powder
- 2 scoops of whey Protein: powder
- 4 eggs
- 2 egg whites
- 1 tablespoon lemon juice
- ¼ cup butter, melted

Directions:

1. Add all the ingredients to the Bread machine.
2. lose the lid and choose Express Bake mode. Once done, take out from the machine and cut into at least 5 pounds.

Nutrition:

- Calories: 257
- Fat: 22.4g
- Carbohydrates: 4.5g
- Protein: 11.5g
- Sodium: 20 mg

Orangey Almond Bacon Bread

Preparation Time: 10 minutes

1-Pound Loaf

Ingredients:

- 1½ cups almond flour
- ½ cup water
- 1 tablespoon baking powder
- 7 oz bacon, diced
- 2 eggs
- 1½ cups cheddar cheese, shredded
- 4 tablespoons butter, melted
- 1/3 cup sour cream

Directions:

1. Add all ingredients to the bread machine.
2. Close the lid and choose the Sweet Bread mode.
3. After the cooking time is over, remove the machine's bread and rest for about 5 minutes.
4. Enjoy!

Nutrition:

- Calories: 307
- Fat: 26 g
- Carbohydrate: 3 g
- Protein: 1 g
- Sodium: 120 mg